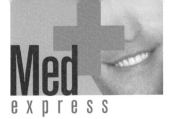

overcoming
colds & flu

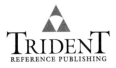

TRIDENT
REFERENCE PUBLISHING

Published by:
Trident Reference Publishing
801 12th Avenue South, Suite 400
Naples, Fl 34102 USA
Phone: + 1 239 649 7077
Email: sales@trident-international.com
Website: www.trident-international.com

Overcoming Colds & Flu
© Trident Reference Publishing

Publisher
Simon St. John Bailey

Editor-in-chief
Isabel Toyos

Art Director
Aline Talavera

Photos
© Trident Reference Publishing, © Getty Images, © Jupiter Images, © Planstock, © J. Alonso

Includes index
ISBN 1582799628 (hc)
UPC 615269996287 (hc)
ISBN 1582799504 (pbk)
UPC 615269995044 (pbk)

2005 Edition
Printed in USA

overcoming colds & flu

 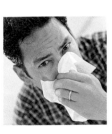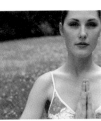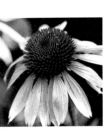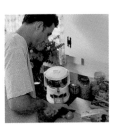

What are respiratory illnesses?

Although they all present similar physical symptoms, the illnesses that attack the respiratory system have very different characteristics and require specific treatments.

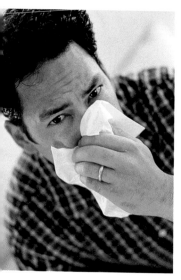

✚ Because respiratory illnesses have such similar symptoms, you should see a doctor to diagnose you correctly. On occasions, when the symptoms first appear you can rest and take an over the counter decongestive medication. However, if symptoms continue, you must seek medical advice.

Staying out in the cold very rarely causes respiratory ailments. In general, they are caused by a viral or bacterial infection. The most common respiratory infections are:

■ **Common chest cold.** Your symptoms include an achy head –especially pains in the ears, nose and throat– sneezing, mucus, cough and sometimes fever.

■ **Flu.** When you come down with the flu, you have an infection in the upper respiratory system. You can catch the flu from viruses in the atmosphere or direct contact with an infected person. The infection hits you suddenly with notorious symptoms such as a sore throat, head ache, tiredness, achy body, loss of appetite, cough and feverish condition. If your symptoms persist for several days, it's important to visit the doctor.

■ **Angina.** You have clear symptoms like intense sore throat that's sometimes accompanied by swollen tonsils, headache and fever. It can be caused by bacteria or viruses and rarely by

mycotic infection.
Other respiratory illnesses:

■ **Tonsillitis** (inflamed tonsils),
laryngitis (inflamed larynx or vocal
cords), **pharyngitis** (inflamed
pharynx). All of these infections
present similar symptoms: fever, sore
throat, headache, cough, phlegm,
chest pressure and difficulty
swallowing and breathing.
■ **Sinusitis** (inflamed sinuses). Pain
or pressure in some areas of the face
(forehead, cheeks or between the eyes), a stuffy
nose, fever and thick green or yellow nasal
mucus can be a sign of sinusitis.
■ **Rhinitis** (inflammation of the lining of the
nose). The symptoms include sneezing and
runny and/or itchy nose.
■ **Bronchitis** (inflammation of the bronchial
tubes). Some of the most common symptoms are
cough, wheezing, fever, and soreness in the chest.
■ **Pleurisy** (inflamed pleura). Generally caused by
an infection in the membranes that cover the
lungs, but it can also be associated with
pneumonia or an infection in another
neighboring organ. When you breathe you have
sharp pains in the chest and shoulders, which are
caused by accumulated liquid in the membranes.
Generally, pleurisy is accompanied by a high fever.
■ **Pneumonia** (infection or inflammation of
the lungs). It can be caused by different micro-
organisms: viruses or bacteria, (but it can also
be caused by corrosive chemicals or toxic
gases). The symptoms of pneumonia develop
abruptly and may include chest pain, fever,
shaking, and chills. It requires immediate
medical care.

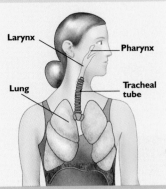

EL SISTEMA RESPIRATORIO

Larynx

Pharynx

Lung

Tracheal
tube

COUGH

*Coughing is a natural
defense mechanism
that our bodies
use to get rid of what
is preventing us from
properly breathing
(dust, smoke). When
you are down
with the flu or suffering
from a respiratory
infection (bronchitis,
laryngitis), coughing
can be very painful.
A cough generally goes
away on its own. But if
you have a cough
for more than two
weeks, chest pains,
fever or if you are
coughing up blood, see a
doctor.*

Fighting colds & flu

When you come down with the first symptoms of a cold, you can rest and take pain relievers. If the symptoms don't go away you should consult a doctor. Natural remedies can also help to relieve symptoms. Holistic treatments should always accompany a medical diagnosis and treatment.

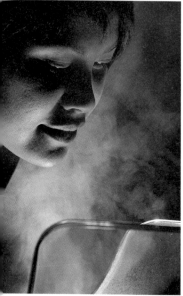

In general, when your symptoms are treated, only if your doctor diagnoses an infection antibiotics should be prescribed. When symptoms become serious, your doctor can take x-rays and other tests to make a more exact diagnosis.

If you have aches, chills and a fever, the best thing to do is to lie down and rest covered up in a warm, well-ventilated room. If the body maintains a fever, it's good to apply a cold washcloth over the face and body, and to rinse off the sweat. It's important to drink plenty of liquids to replace salt and minerals you lose when you sweat. Unlike babies, who should receive immediate medical attention and be administered anti-fever medication and lukewarm baths, adults should consult their physician before taking medication.

ANTIBIOTICS

You should never take antibiotics without a medical prescription. Once you start taking antibiotics it is fundamental to complete the treatment. Always take them for the complete period prescribed by your doctor, even if you start to feel better or if the symptoms go away.

The idea is to avoid getting rid of the symptoms, for your doctor to be able to use them in a proper diagnosis of the illness.

One of the first symptoms of a **cold** may be excessive thirst. This is a result of the increased calories that your body burns to fight the infection. It's recommended to drink plenty of cold water and to avoid drinking tea, coffee or soft drinks. If you come down with the **flu** you should rest and treat your symptoms. However, if you don't feel better after 3 or 4 days, you should see a doctor.

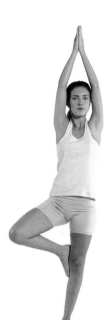

A doctor, who can determine whether there are bacteria in the throat, should always treat **angina**. If the test comes out positive, it's generally treated with antibiotics. **Tonsillitis, laryngitis, bronchitis** are all infections treated with rest, vapors, and pain relievers, but if symptoms persist for more than 2 days you should see a doctor.

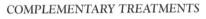

COMPLEMENTARY TREATMENTS

- *Yoga.*
- *Shiatsu.*
- *Reflexology.*
- *Hydrotherapy.*
- *Using essential oils in aromatherapy.*
- *Using medicinal herbs in infusions and inhalations.*
- *Nutritional and dietary therapy.*

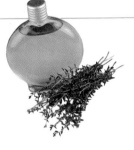

A physician should treat **pleurisy**. Along with prescribed medication, you should get plenty of rest and drink a lot of fluids. Hot compresses applied to the back and chest can also help to alleviate symptoms and help you to get better. With these illnesses, you should avoid sudden changes of temperature, use disposable tissues and wash your hands often.

Yoga to improve breathing

Yoga is a technique dating back thousands of years. Its principles are based on creating harmony between the mind, body and spirit. Regularly practicing yoga can help to relieve and fight colds, flu, bronchitis and other respiratory ailments because the exercises lay on teaching you to relax and to breath better.

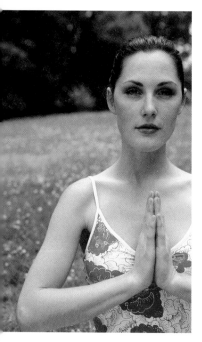

Yoga originated in India and dates back more than 5,000 years. Yoga is considered a philosophy, science, art and therapy that aims to attain the unity of mind, body and spirit through the teaching of body postures, breathing, relaxation, concentration and meditation.

The word "yoga" means to unite or to join together our potential to reach a balance between our spiritual, mental and physical state. The discipline aims to develop our mental awareness and to identify the energy that flows inside of our bodies and the Universe using this force to improve our stamina and health, to awaken our spirit and to connect our bodies to the Universe's energy.

Each yoga pose (also known as *asana*) is thought to improve your body's functions –brain, cells, muscles, glands, organs, nerves and tissues– while at the same time increasing your clarity and mental concentration. The poses also prepare the body and mind for meditation, a state that brings serenity and union between the body, the mind and the spirit and the Universe.

HOW TO GET READY

Before practicing yoga postures or *asanas*, you should prepare your body through a series of stretching exercises to warm up your muscles and to release tension. It's best to do these poses on a padded mat or carpeted floor, which will help you to feel more comfortable and confident, and prevent you from hitting your body on a hard surfaced floor.

Rocking chair

This pose, called the Rocking chair or Hammock, is good for loosening and toning your muscles.

I. Sit on the floor, with your chin pressed against your chest. Bend your legs, with your feet on the floor and your hands behind your thighs.

2. Bring your torso backward to the floor, lifting your legs up and supporting them with your arms to continue to bring your legs back.

3. With the same motion, bring your legs back until they touch the floor. Next, bring them up, taking care not to lift up your chin. Continue the exercise, bringing your legs back and then forward at least 7 times continuously, without taking a rest between the sets.

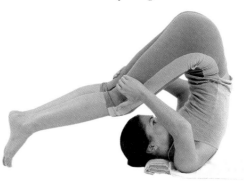

THE IMPORTANCE OF BREATHING

Because of its deep purifying effects on the respiratory system, exercising the breath when practicing yoga helps you to manage respiratory ailments like asthma and bronchitis by removing mucus.

Breathing exercises help you achieve a calm and alert mind. Throughout time we become aware of the process of breathing and discover the capacity that our lungs have. To increase your overall health and to prevent and cure respiratory illnesses, it's best to practice complete yoga sessions at least two times per week. These exercises or poses can be practiced at any time, although it's best to do them in the morning before starting your day.

Basic breathing techniques

Practicing breathing is a fundamental element in yoga. From the start, it's important to concentrate on the differences in your body when you are tense or relaxed, and when you are resting or using your body. There is a strong relationship between your emotional state and your breathing. Practicing yoga helps you to become conscious of the respiratory process. Over time and with effort, you will learn to improve your physical and mental health through breathing. Taking deep breaths, for example, changes your mental and physical state and makes you feel better. This is what is called "complete breathing" consisting of three types of breathing: abdominal, thoracic and clavicular.

■ Abdominal or diaphragmatic breathing

This is the easiest breathing technique. Lie down on the floor and rest both hands on your abdomen.

A SMART TIP
When you first begin these exercises it may be difficult for you to make sure that you expand your abdomen. To find out if you are doing this exercise properly, place a book on your abdomen. You will see the book rises as you inhale and then slowly descends as you exhale.

Take a deep breath, inhaling slowly through your nose, expanding the abdomen voluntarily, concentrating your energy in that spot. Hold your breath for a few seconds. Then slowly exhale, contracting your abdomen.

■ Thoracic breathing

In the same position, place your hands over the middle parts of the lungs and concentrate on the energy in this area. Without moving your abdomen, take a deep breath and note how your ribs rise and your chest expands as the air enters. Next, slowly exhale, thinking about how your thoracic box closes.

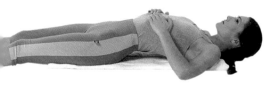

■ Clavicular or collarbone breathing

Using the same position, place your hands on your chest or on the collarbone. Inhale and exhale through the nose, paying attention to how it feels when the air lifts your ribs, collarbone and shoulders. (The body does not take in sufficient oxygen with this type of breathing, so it's best not to practice this exercise for very long.)

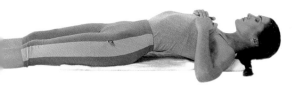

COMPLETE BREATHING

Complete breathing is a combination of clavicular breathing, thoracic breathing and abdominal breathing. The exercise involves the entire respiratory system to increase your lungs capacity and to relax your body and mind. First, inhale and expand your abdomen, then your thorax and finally your upper chest. Exhale in the same order, first contracting your abdomen, then your thorax and finally your upper chest.

THE PRANAYAMA

Yoga is the belief and practice which aims to extend the breathing process to absorb and distribute the vital life energy (also known as *prana*).

The *Pranayama* is a technique used to regulate the process of breathing. This technique is based on the yogi philosophy or study of the relationship between body and mind. It is recommended that you begin practicing *Pranayama* at least 6 months after initiating the *asana* exercises.

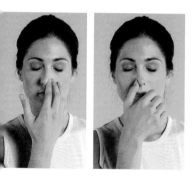

The Alternate nostril breathing
(*Nadi shodhana pranayama*)
Helps to normalize the breathing cycle and can be done in any comfortable *asana* pose. The technique is done by alternately breathing through each of the nostrils. Begin by closing one nostril with your fingers and breathing 10 rounds. Breathe 10 rounds on each side. Over time you can slowly increase the rhythm. However, never force your breath.

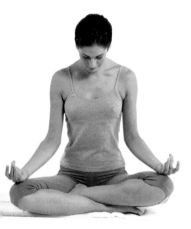

The Cleansing breath
(*Kapalabhati pranayama*)
Kapalabhati is a breathing technique used specifically for cleansing. It's a good exercise for smokers to use to detoxify the lungs. In the Lotus position or sitting with your legs crossed, begin by taking 10 quick breaths, and when you exhale pull in your abdomen (it's normal that when the air is expelled through the nose it makes more sound than you're accustomed to).

Complete three sets of 10 breaths, although a *Kapalabhati* session can be more complete. When you end a set, inhale deeply and exhale fully. Next, with your lungs filled with air, lower the head to close your airway, tensing your buttocks and forming a *mudra* with your hands. Stay in this position as long as you comfortably can, but without straining yourself. Lastly, before exhaling, bring your head facing forward, release your buttocks and move out of the position.

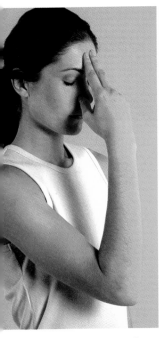

NASAGRA MUDRA

(*Nasagra*) This breathing technique can improve nasal breathing. Place the tips of your index and middle fingers on your forehead. Your thumb should be on your right side and your pinkie and ring fingers on your left side. Start by breathing, alternating nostrils, by closing the nostril one side at a time. The contact of your fingers on your forehead stimulates your *ajna chakra*, better known as the "third eye" that is believed to bring greater mental insight, self-control, clairvoyance, superior intuition and extrasensorial perception.

THE SUN SALUTATION OR SURYA NAMASKAR

This is a graceful sequence of twelve yoga positions performed as one continuous exercise. This exercise is good for the respiratory system and beneficial for other parts of the body.

The Sun Salutation limbers up the whole body in preparation for the yoga *asana* postures because it uses the spinal column, arms and legs. If practiced daily this pose will increase your body's stamina and blood circulation, while balancing the respiratory, digestive and nervous systems. It improves the flexibility of your spine and joints and trims your waist. It also helps to prevent back pains and improves the body's posture.

GENTLE EXERCISE

Yoga is a discipline designed to improve your flexibility and harmony. The exercises use gentle movements without straining your body. When practicing the *asanas* remember not to strain yourself. There is no need to push yourself too far. Throughout time and willpower, you will improve your body's health naturally and get in tune with your body.

1. To begin the Surya namaskar or Sun Salutation (which is considered one of the most complete yoga exercises) stand on your feet, with your back straight, ankles together and buttocks tight. Bring your hands to the chest with the palms together, take a deep breath and hold your breath in for a moment. Next, exhale.

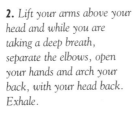

2. Lift your arms above your head and while you are taking a deep breath, separate the elbows, open your hands and arch your back, with your head back. Exhale.

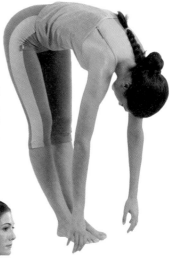

3. Bend your body forward without bending the knees. Relax your neck and touch the floor with your hands.

4. In a squatting position, take in a deep breath and extend your left leg back, bending your right knee into your chest. Exhale, with your arms to the sides of your body.

5. With your hands on the floor, extend your right leg backward also and put the weight of your legs on your toes, with your ankles together and your arms stretched out.

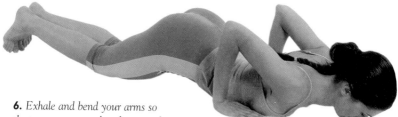

6. Exhale and bend your arms so that your torso touches the ground, keeping your hips elevated for a few seconds. Your body's weight should be distributed between your chin, chest and knees.

7. Inhale and lean on the lower part of your body, while you lift up your chest and shoulders and bend your head backward, with your eyes closed.

8. Placing on the palms of your hands and the soles of your feet on the ground, lift your hips up and make a bridge, with your legs straight and your head relaxed (the Tent position).

9. Repeat step 4, this time with your right leg back and your left knee bent into the chest.

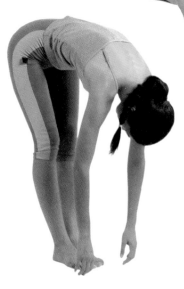

10. Repeat step 3 (torso lowered, head relaxed, legs straight and touching the floor with your hands). Stay in this position for a few seconds.

11. Inhale, lift up your body and repeat step 2 (head backward, back arched and arms extended upward).

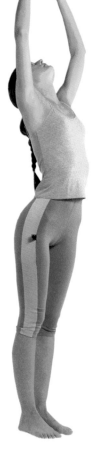

FINAL POSITION

Return to the first position, with your back straight and your hands with palms together on your chest. The philosophy of yoga considers that this hand position means peace between body, mind, spirit and Universe.

The poses

Yoga poses or *asanas* aim to strengthen and balance the body. Some *asanas* are especially good for harmonizing and facilitating proper breathing, preventing lung and bronchial disorders and relieving the symptoms of respiratory illnesses.

The Fish

The Fish yoga pose can help complications related to asthma and bronchitial ailments, because it exercises and expands the chest muscles. Also it tones the back and abdominal muscles.

1. Sit with your back straight and your buttocks resting on your heels. Place your hands, palms down, on your thighs.

2. Breathing freely, bring your head all the way back, arching your back and leaning your elbows and hands on the floor.

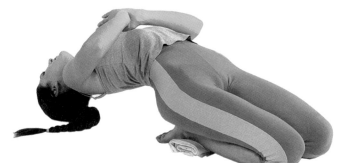

3. *Drop your head back so that the top of your head is on the floor, but your weight should rest on your elbows. Exhale. Bring your hands to your chest, with the palms together, stay in this position as long as you can. Next, inhale and place your elbows on the floor, bring your chin to your chest. Come out of the pose by rolling onto your side.*

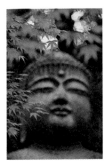

BRANCHES OF YOGA

There are different types of yoga, although they all have the same objective.

• **Hatha yoga:** *is the path of physical yoga and is the most popular branch of yoga. It uses physical poses or asanas, breathing techniques (or pranayamas), energy flows (bandas) and psychic gestures (mudras).*

• **Raja yoga:** *is the path of yoga that focuses on meditation and contemplation.*

• **Karma yoga:** *believes that your present situation is based on your past actions. The pillars are good words, good thoughts and good deeds.*

• **Jnana yoga:** *is the path of yoga that deals with wisdom and knowledge or the yoga of the mind.*

• **Bhaki yoga:** *is the path of heart and devotion, to see the Divine in everyone and everything he or she encounters.*

YOGA AND MEDICINE

Over the past years, Western medicine has begun to accept the medical benefits of this thousand year old technique and has adopted yoga and the general lifestyle change involved in it. Unlike Western medicine, which is largely based on a science of disease and treatment, yoga is a science of health. The teachings of yoga are based on an intricate and precise understanding of the healthy functioning of the human body and mind. Its techniques are designed to maximize your own potential for good health, vitality and lasting youthfulness.

The Candle

This pose is helpful in accompanying the treatment of asthma and bronchitis. It also improves blood circulation and helps to prevent varicose veins.

1. Lying down, inhale, extend your arms next to your body, and lift your legs until they form a 90 degree angle. Exhale and when you inhale again lift up your hips and back, bringing your legs over your head.

2. Bend your arms, keep your hands on your back and bring your feet to the floor. Raise your left leg, stretched (your chin needs to be pressed against your chest, so that your neck doesn't tense up).

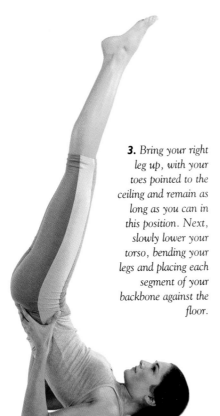

3. Bring your right leg up, with your toes pointed to the ceiling and remain as long as you can in this position. Next, slowly lower your torso, bending your legs and placing each segment of your backbone against the floor.

GOOD NEWS

As an example of the importance yoga has gained in the medical field, this exercise is being used as a treatment in carpal tunnel syndrome. Carpal tunnel syndrome occurs when the median nerve, which runs from the forearm into the hand, becomes pressed or squeezed at the wrist, causing pain. This condition is associated with those who work on a keyboard or repetitive activities that strain the wrist. Surgical treatment can be used, but not on all patients.

THE LION'S ROAR

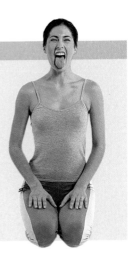

- This is a very particular *asana* because it is centered around a muscle that is seldom used in traditional exercises: the tongue. This pose not only stretches the tongue, it also helps to relieve sore throats and to prevent tonsillitis and pharyngitis.
- Sit with your buttocks on your heels, back straight and hands on your thighs. Inhale and relax your jaw, stick out your tongue and exhale through the nose. Each time you exhale, stick out your tongue more as if you were trying to touch your chin with it.

Renewing shiatsu

Shiatsu is a traditional Asian technique involving finger pressure to bring your life energy into harmony. *Shiatsu* sessions benefit the flow of air in the body and the fight against respiratory infections.

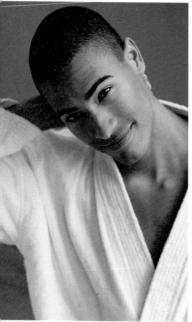

✚ *Shiatsu* originated over 6,000 years ago as a teaching of Chinese medicine. The technique wasn't introduced to the rest of the world until the middle of the 20th century.

Shi means "fingers" and *atsu* means "pressure". *Shiatsu* means "finger pressure" in Japanese. The technique is also called Japanese finger acupressure. Using the rhythmic pressing of acupressure points for short periods, the *shiatsu* technique is a treatment that works on the meridians of the body to put our *chi* or life energy in balance. This energy can be either yin or yang (passive-active, negative-positive).

The organs can also be yin or yang. The *chi* or vital energy should flow harmonically through the organs. When the flow is unbalanced it produces ailments.

The philosophy underlying *shiatsu* considers that if we eat a healthy diet, breath correctly and maintain a strong and flexible body the *chi* flows freely, bringing good health.

As with other holistic remedies, *shiatsu* aims to increase our immune system's ability to cure illnesses in the body by stimulating the flow

of the *chi*. *Shiatsu* sessions are an
excellent treatment for coughs,
common colds and asthma.

■ **Nasal congestion and headache.**
This massage helps to relieve nasal
congestion and headaches. Begin by
pinching the eyebrows with the index
finger and thumb of both of your
hands, starting in the center and then
moving toward the temples. Repeat
this massage several times.

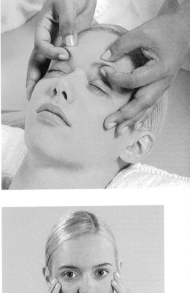

■ **Colds.**
A good way to relieve cold symptoms
which are making you feel bad is to
gently press with your fingertips the
area around the eyes.

■ **Sinus infections and the flu.**
Press with your index and middle
fingers on both sides of the nose to
help relieve sinus pains caused by
sinus infections and the flu.

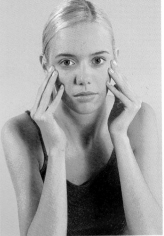

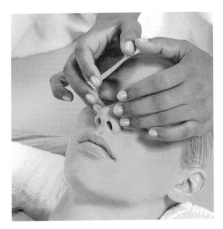

Strengthening reflexology

Reflexology has been used as a natural healing art for thousands of years in China, Malaysia and India. The technique helps overall health and relieves aches and pains by applying pressure on the edges and base of the feet, toes and hands. Reflexology can help to prevent the flu and to relieve respiratory problems.

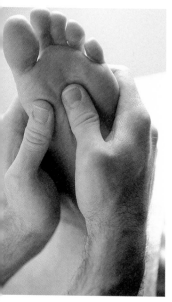

This natural healing art is based on the principle and study that there are reflexes in the body –especially in the feet and hands– that correspond to the body's organs and glands. Applying stimulation and pressure to the feet or hands, can affect the health of other parts of the body. Modern reflexology is based on the work of US physician William Fitzgerald, who in the early 20th century developed the ancient Oriental healing art of using pressure to relieve pains into a usable diagnostic therapy.

Reflexology is not an exact science, but has been proven through practice to give positive results. You don't need to be a specialist to give these relaxing massages, you can practice them with someone else or on yourself.

The following massages are a good way to fight stress and to stimulate blood flow to the affected organs. There are specific massages to help alleviate excess mucus, headaches, coughs and other symptoms brought on by colds, flu and bronchitis.

ON THE HANDS

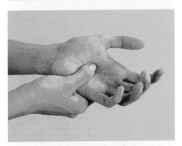

There are also reflex points on the hands. The following exercise is the perfect massage or self-massage to provide relief for headaches.

With the index finger and thumb, massage the soft part of the palm of your hand, applying firm pressure with the two fingers and concentrating on the side of the hand that corresponds to where your pain is coming from.

Pregnant women should avoid this exercise, because it is the same reflex point to stimulate giving birth.

IMPORTANT

For colds, flu and bronchitis, it's good to give yourself a massage to release tension and to increase sensibility in the feet. This will help to more accurately stimulate pressure points on the bottom and edges of the feet, focusing on the most important points such as the head, eyes, ears, throat, and lungs, as indicated in the diagram.

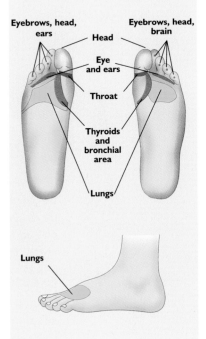

Eyebrows, head, ears — Head — Eyebrows, head, brain — Eye and ears — Throat — Thyroids and bronchial area — Lungs — Lungs

HEADACHES

To treat headaches there are specific massages on the feet.

Start by using firm circular movements with your thumb on your big toe, which will help to loosen the neck. Next, apply strong pressure over the reflex areas that correspond to the head (see above diagrams), using your thumb.

ON THE FEET

ASTHMA AND BRONCHITIS
Reflexology can be very useful in the treatment of asthma, bronchitis and smokers' cough. Using your fingertips, apply steady, penetrating pressure to the points that correspond to the lungs.

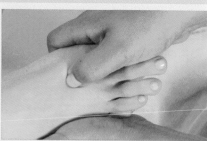

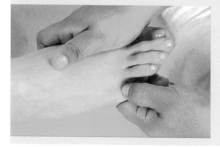

EARACHES
To relief earaches apply pressure to the points on the foot that correspond to the ears, behind the toes.

This pressure can cause you some discomfort, but you should continue with the massage and the discomfort will pass. Continue applying pressure with your thumb lower and on the tip of your big toe.

SAFETY
Although reflexology is not an aggressive treatment, it can present side effects with certain conditions: pregnancy (especially if there is risk of miscarriage), fever, serious diseases, problems that require emergency surgery, gangrene, injuries or foot conditions, and serious infections.

EXCESS MUCUS

When you have a cold or cough and a lot of mucus and pressure in the sinus area, massaging the areas that correspond to the suprarenal gland and the ileac valve can help you feel better.

COMMON COLD

To treat a cold with reflexology it's good to apply pressure to all of the reflex areas that correspond to the head. Concentrate the pressure to the points that correspond to the nose, throat, lungs, eyes, ears and the sinuses.

WHAT IS A REFLEXOLOGY SESSION LIKE?

Normally a reflexology session lasts for half an hour, depending on the sensibility of the feet. One session per week is recommended when beginning treatment, although you can decide how often you use reflexology depending on your needs.

- *A session begins with a deep cleansing of the feet.*

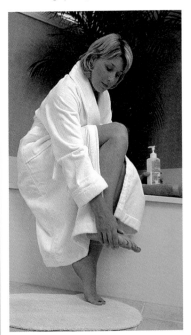

- *Next, try to clear your mind by closing your eyes, thinking nice thoughts and breathing through the nose deeply at least three times.*
- *To get your muscles ready, the practitioner will massage the entire sole of your foot and your ankle. Then the reflexologist will roll your ankle and gently massage each toe.*
- *The practitioner will then ask you what problems you are having and examine each foot. This is done in order to know what pressure points to work on. The reflexologist will press on each of the reflex points, one by one.*
- *The body is divided into ten longitudinal zones, five zones on each side. The organ in that specific zone will correspond to that same longitudinal zone on the foot.*
- *The stimulating pressure can be very comforting, nevertheless stimulating some pressure points can cause discomfort. This response will help the practitioner find corporal imbalances and design a suitable massage session to treat them.*
- *Sessions can be so relaxing that some patients might fall asleep, while others might feel energized and rejuvenated. It's best to follow what your body feels and needs, whether it is to move around or rest.*
- *In general, reflexology doesn't present any side-effects. However, when begining treatment some patients may feel as if symptoms get worse. This is known as "crisis when curing". Crisis occurs when the process of detoxifying takes place in the body. You don't need to worry, this is a good sign, it means that the treatment is working effectively on your body.*

Soothing hydrotherapy

Hydrotherapy is the use of water at different temperatures to revitalize, maintain, and restore health. It is an effective therapy for many ailments, including colds and flu.

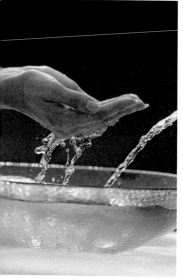

Ancient Greeks and Roman used sources of water for their healing properties, but later the practice was lost. By the 18th and 19th centuries, the method of using water therapeutically was readopted and introduced as a medical treatment. Hydrotherapy is used to stimulate our bodies' internal activity, which helps our bodies' immune systems, but also in the prevention and treatment of illnesses.

Common hydrotherapy techniques are:
• Soaking and rubbing, that may increase blood circulation and regulate breathing.
• Hot and cold compresses, may help to lower fevers and to stimulate blood flow.
• Cold Showers and cold baths, may stimulate the circulatory and nervous systems.
• Hot showers and hot baths may help you to relax.
• Shower streams aimed at a specific affected part of the body.
• Sauna and steam baths, which may help to relieve congestion.

IMMEDIATE REFLIEF

There are specific hydrotherapy treatments for congestion and chills that also may help to release toxins in the body and reduce your susceptibility to illnesses.

Prevention

- Taking a cold bath for 10 minutes may help your immune system to prevent colds and to increase your energy, only if you are accustomed to taking cold baths. When you get out of the bath tub, its best to exercise or rest covered up, cozy in bed.
- The healing therapies of water can be intensified by adding cider vinegar or sea salts (calculate 1 cup of vinegar per bathtub, or 2 teaspoons of sea salt for every 33 fl oz/1 liter of water).

For cases of colds and fevers

- With the first signs of a cold, it may be helpful to soak in a warm bath (it's best to stay in the bathtub no longer than 20 minutes). Compresses moistened with cold water are very good for lowering fevers, especially for children. Place a compress on the forehead and change it every 10 minutes or whenever the linen cloth begins to warm up. You can also use compresses on other parts of the body, such as the underarms, chest and behind the knees.
- In the case of a high fever, doctors may recommend a lukewarm bath. When you get out it's important to cover up with a dry towel and then go to bed, covered up.
- For congested respiratory tracts steam baths can be very effective. Close the bath room door, turn on the faucet for hot water and wait until the bathroom fills up with steam. Stay in the steam bathroom for at least 5 minutes. This treatment may be very useful for relieving children when they are fighting against a stuffed up nose.

ANTI-FEVER HYDRATION
Drinking a lot of fresh water at room temperature and lukewarm teas can be good for fevers and for fighting colds and infections such as angina.

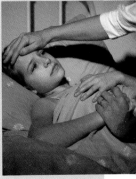

WATER AND SALT GARGLE
Gargling with salt water can work as a great remedy to relieve a sore throat. To prepare, add 1 teaspoon of salt to 1 glass of lukewarm water.

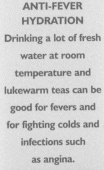

Healing herbs and essential oils

Medical plants can help to treat respiratory infections like the flu, colds and bronchitis. Essential oils (listed in the box alphabetically) are made from highly concentrated essences of plants that have similar health benefits as herbal remedies but are used in aromatherapy.

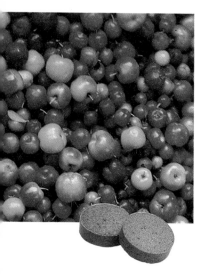

The following are effective medical plants and herbal remedies to fight respiratory ailments. Some plants may be easier to find than others depending on where the plants are cultivated. You can find some as fresh or dried plants, and others in liquid form, tablets or powder.

Acerola or Barbados cherry
(*Malpighia glabra*)

• **Parts used.** The fruit is similar to the common cherry because of its size and color. The fruit is harvested in the summer and eaten fresh. The fruit can also be consumed as capsules, gels or juices.

• Every $1/2$ cup of acerola pulp contains between $1/2$ to 1 teaspoon

NOTE
You should always consult your physician before starting any herbal treatment.

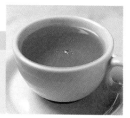

ANTI-FLU INFUSION
Mix 2 tablespoons of acerola with 1 tablespoon of orange peel. Mix 2 teaspoons of this mixture with 1 cup of boiling water. Let it steep, strain and drink a cup $1/2$ hour before eating lunch.

of ascorbic acid or vitamin C (50 to 100 times more than citrus fruit).

• The plant is native to the Yucatan, Mexico. Today, it is cultivated in sub-tropical areas throughout the world, mostly in Brazil. It has a sweet and sour taste.

• It helps to prevent and treat common colds, especially for children and women who are pregnant or breast-feeding. Vitamin C in elevated doses (as with acerola) can help to cure the flu, colds and pulmonary infections.

• Recommended intake for a 1 year old is 1 fruit per day; 10 years of age and older, 2 fruits per day.

• **Warning.** Vitamin C is not recommended for kidney stone sufferers or for those undergoing chemotherapy.

Avenca

(Adiantum capillus-veneris)

• **Parts used.** The leaves are used to prepare in gels, teas and infusions. Avenca is a fern widely used in holistic medicine that grows in moist, covered areas.

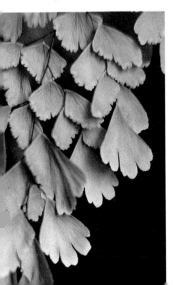

• Native to Europe and Asia, it is widely cultivated in South America.

• It helps as an anti-flu and anti-cold remedy. Good for fighting coughs, bronchitis, sore throats and chronic running nose.

ESSENTIAL OILS FROM A TO Z

BASIL

Basil carries special antiviral, antiseptic, antispasmodic and antibacterial properties. When used on the body it can purify and detoxify the skin. It's recommended diluting basil oil when using it to massage.

Safety. Prolonged use can irritate the skin.

BENJUI

Anti-flu and anti-septic remedy from the Sumatra region. The resin from the plant's gum is used to make an essential oil. It is used in ointments, lotions and creams. Benjui helps to soothe sore throats and is an ideal remedy for children. It's recommended applying a few drops to the affected area.

WARNING

Essential oils are for external use **only**, they should **never** be ingested. Keep stored away from children and keep away from your eyes.

FOR CHILDREN WITH COUGHS
To relieve coughs in children, boil a handful of avenca leaves until the water becomes paste like. Drain and add 2 cups of sugar; allowing the drained mixture to boil for a few more minutes. Take 2 to 3 spoonfuls a day. Avenca can also be prepared as an infusion and drunk through a filtered straw.

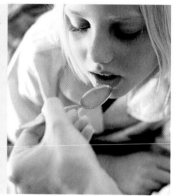

AROMATHERAPY

Although modern aromatherapy is thought of as a technique to care for the body with pleasant smells, this ancient healing art uses essential oils for their therapeutic properties. Essential oils are extracted from plants, flowers, trees, and roots and processed

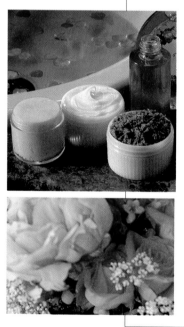

by grinding, distillation, or extracted with a dissolvent. Essential oils can be diluted and mixed with other vegetable-based oils because they tend to be costly and very concentrated.

Some uses for essential oils: rub into skin during massages, put a few drops when taking a bath and add to vapors for inhaling. Essential oils should be ingested only under strict medical supervision. Using oils in massage therapy is the most common use because it awakens the sense of smell, softens the skin and makes the massage feel even more relaxing.

Essential oils are good for use in treating respiratory ailments (see Essential oils from A to Z box, on page 31).

Ephedra or Ma Huang

(Ephedra sinica)

• **Parts used.** The stems are used to make powders and tinctures. In India ephedra is used as the principle component in soma, a potent tonic. Ephedra's main active medicinal ingredient is the alkaloid ephedrine, which is used to treat asthma.

• The Chinese have used ephedra medicinally for over 5,000 years as a natural remedy to treat serious illnesses, including asthma and lung and bronchial constriction.

• Ephedra is good for moving mucus and fluids, fighting the chills, headaches, aches and pains and coughs.

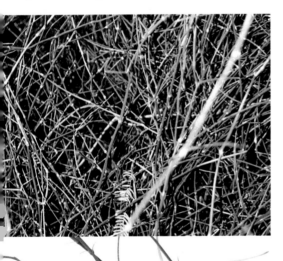

• **Safety.** Ephedra should not be used with symptoms of high blood pressure or if you are taking other stimulants or anti-depressive drugs. In some nations, law controls the maximum dosage. Efedrine is also included in a list of drugs banned in professional sports.

Echinacea
(*Echinacea purpurea*)

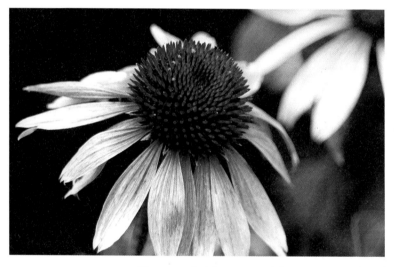

• **Parts used.** The root and flowers are used. Echinacea powder and tincture are made from the plant's roots. Relatively recently, the flowers began to be used to make capsules.

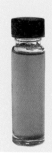

NATURAL COUGH SYRUP
Take $^1/_2$ spoonful of echinacea tincture with water 2 or 3 times a day to relieve a dry chest cough and bronchitis.

• Echinacea is a wild flower native to North America. Native Americans used the plant for a variety of conditions, including high fevers and venomous bites. The colonists adopted echinacea as a home remedy against colds and flu. In the past decades its use has expanded throughout the globe for its antiviral and antibacterial properties.

• It can be administered to children for sore throats. Add 2 teaspoons of root tincture to a glass of tepid water and gargle.

• **Safety** (especially for taking orally as a tincture or a concoction). Large doses can cause nausea and dizziness. It shouldn't be used if you have autoimmune illnesses.

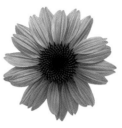

Eucalyptus
(Eucalyptus globulus)

• **Parts used.** The leaves are cultivated all year long. They can be used to make infusions and also for capsules and pills. Infusions are recommended for children (you can sweeten them with honey).

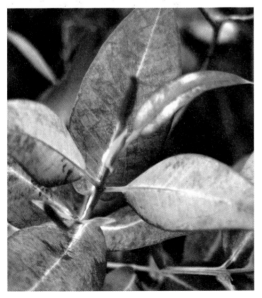

ESSENTIAL OILS FROM **A** TO **Z**

CEDAR
Calming and antiseptic, which is useful for treating respiratory illnesses. It was one of the first oils to be used as a healing remedy; the ancient Egyptians used cedar oil to cure throat ailments. Native Americans have for centuries considered cedar trees as sacred for their healing properties.

CINNAMON
Anti-fever. Cinnamon has a warm, sweet and spicy aroma, which is a good remedy for high fevers accompanied by chills. However, it's best to use cinnamon oil in low concentrates. Take care when using the oil made from the tree's leaves. The bark is used exclusively for the skin.

KIDS SUFFERING FROM A COLD

To relieve nasal congestion, place 1 drop of lavender oil and a drop of eucalyptus oil on a handkerchief and place under the pillow for a night.

• Eucalyptus is native to Australia, where aboriginal natives used the plant as a remedy against fever. During the 14th century the plant was introduced to Europe and today it is grown across America and Europe.

• This remedy fights against the flu virus and other bacteriae. It also has antiseptic properties because of its high cineol content. The leaves are ground to make capsules that are a remedy for respiratory infections and bronchitis.

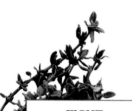

FIGHT BRONCHITIS

Mix 5 drops of eucalyptus, 5 of thyme with 2 spoonfuls of olive or sunflower oil. Rub this mixture into the chest or back, 2 times a day. **Safety.** Do not use thyme essential oil during pregnancy.

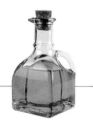

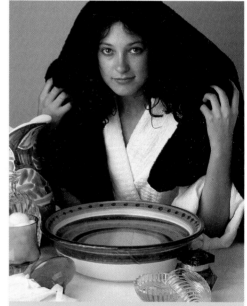

VAPOR FOR PULMONARY AILMENTS

Place 10 drops of eucalyptus oil in a bowl with water at the point of boiling. Cover the head and take deep breaths with the vapor for 15 minutes.

Coltsfoot
(Tussilago farfara)

- **Parts used.** The leaves and flowers are cultivated at the end of spring.
- Native to central Europe, it is cultivated as a medicinal plant.
- Coltsfoot may be used in chronic or acute bronchitis, irritating coughs, whooping coughs and asthma. Its soothing expectorant action gives coltsfoot a role in most respiratory conditions.
- **Warning.** It's best to avoid coltsfoot during pregnancy and breast-feeding. It shouldn't be used as a prolonged treatment; or for those who have liver troubles.

TO CONTROL YOUR COUGH
To soothe an irritating cough, use 2 tablespoons coltsfoot leaves or flowers for every 4 cups of water. Boil for 5 minutes and strain to make a tea. Drink 3 cups a day.

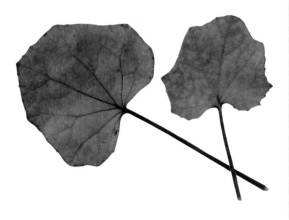

ESSENTIAL OILS FROM A TO Z

CYPRUS
Antispasmodic. When used in a vapor, this oil helps to soothe respiratory problems. It is anti-septic, refreshing and soothing. It's used for snoring and sore throat. It's inhaled for sore throats and convulsive coughs. It's used in cases of epilepsy.

EUCALYPTUS
A powerful antiseptic that helps respiratory infections and asthma. It helps to decongest stuffed up noses and to relieve sore throats and coughs. It's used in massages, scrubbings, compresses and vapor treatment. It's a powerful oil, so it should be used in lower concentration, especially when used on children. It mixes well with lavender.

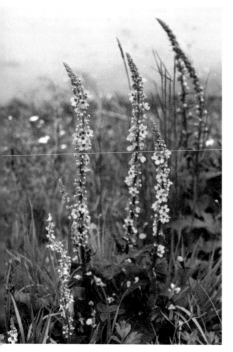

Mullein
(Verbascum thapsus)

• **Parts used.** The flowers. The bright yellow flowers are used fresh, dried or ground to make infusions. The fruit is also used to fight respiratory problems for its soothing emollient properties.

• The plant can grow up to two meters high. Although its origin is unknown, it was used in Mexico before the Spanish conquest.

• The plant is an excellent remedy for soothing and calming the bronchial tubes, and to relieve continual and irritating coughs.

• **Warning.** Mullein shouldn't be used during pregnancy and breastfeeding.

OCCASIONAL SORE THROAT

Take a handful of fresh English ivy leaves, wash them and let them dry. Next, grind them with a mortar to extract the plant's liquid.
Place 1 tablespoon of the zest in 2 cups of water and let rest for 10 minutes. Drink this mixture (3 cups per day) sweetened with honey. English ivy blends well with elderberry flowers and with plantain: use 2 parts English ivy for 1 part of the other two herbs.

SOAK IN AN ANTI-COLD BATH
Soak in a bath with 5 drops of fennel oil to help relieve a persistent congestion.

TO RELIEVE EXCESS MUCUS
Mix 1 teaspoon of essential oil of fennel with 1 tablespoon of neutral oil as an ointment to rub on the chest.

English Ivy
(Hedera helyx)

• **Parts used.** Fresh leaves and dried leaves and flowers, to grind into powder, to make tonics and infusions.

• English ivy is native to Central Europe and was used widely in the Middle Ages.

• English ivy has soothing, antiseptic and astringent properties; it helps to dry up mucus in the bronchial tubes and to clear up stuffed up sinuses. Taken as a tonic or infusion, it's good for sore throats, stuffy noses and upper respiratory ailments. It also helps to relieve sinus infections.

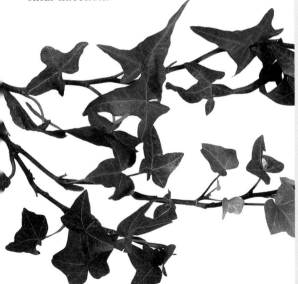

ESSENTIAL OILS FROM A TO Z

EUFRASIA

Antitusive and anti-cold remedy, it's also known for its antiseptic properties. The parts of the plant growing above the ground are used to make vapors and ointments for massages.
Safety. It shouldn't be used for children under 2 years old.

FENNEL

This essential oil is soothing and it also has antiseptic properties. It's used in massages, compresses and vapor treatment to clear up bronchial mucus.
It can be blended with marsh mallow and thyme.
Safety. This oil shouldn't be used for prolonged periods without alternating between other oils. It shouldn't be used on pregnant women or those who suffer from epilepsy.

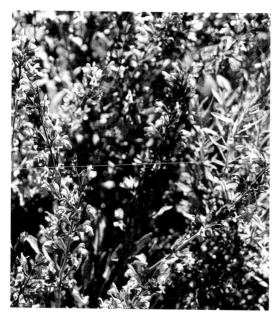

Hyssop
(*Hysopus officinalis*)

• **Parts used.**
The stems and flowers are used in tinctures and capsules as a remedy to sooth bronchitis. It has a spicy aroma that blends well with thyme and basil.
• This shrub is native to the Mediterranean, but it is also grown in Central Europe and Western Asia.
• Hyssop's bitter and spicy taste has a tonic and stimulating effect on the respiratory system. It's also good for soothing a sore throat and persistent cough. This remedy helps to stimulate sweating if you have the chills or flu. It blends well with liquorice (*glycyrhiza glabra*) to relieve bronchitis and a chronic cough.
• **Warning.** Avoid use during pregnancy and for those with epilepsy. You should never exceed the recommended dose, because this essential oil can provoke seizures.

ESSENTIAL OILS FOR RESPIRATORY PROBLEMS
Mix 1 drop of myrrh, 1 drop lavender and 1 drop of orange in 2 tablespoons of neutral oil or cream. You can use this soothing ointment to rub on the chest or back.

FOR EARACHES

Ideal remedy for children
Place 2 drops of lavender oil on cotton balls and place them in the ears until the pain goes away

Ginger
(Zingiber officinalis)

• **Parts used.** The roots are used fresh or dehydrated.
• This zesty tasting root, native to India and China, is currently grown throughout the world.
• Ginger is a good anti-flu remedy because it has 12 antiviral components. It helps to relieve symptoms that accompany colds, fevers and aches. It also soothes cough and helps you to rest. Also, it's an excellent emetic. Ginger can be taken in a tea, or in infusions or capsules that are made with the root.
• **Warning.** It's not recommended for prolonged use during pregnancy. Do not use this remedy if you are taking blood-clotting drugs.

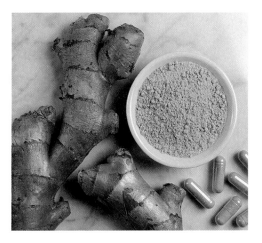

ESSENTIAL OILS FROM A TO Z

LAVENDER
Antibiotic and sedative that helps to fight sinus infections and ailments caused by the common cold such as exhaustion, headaches and earaches. This oil adapts well on all types of skin. To relieve flu or cold symptoms massage on the cheekbones and sinuses.
Safety. Do not use this oil during the first three months of pregnancy. If you have low blood pressure lavender can cause drowsiness.

LEMON HERB
This anti-flu, antiseptic and antibacterial remedy is useful in soothing a sore throat and to lower a fever. It is a strong oil and should be diluted to avoid skin irritation. It blends well with essential oils of basil, cedar, eucalyptus, geranium, lavender, tea tree and rosemary.
Safety. Avoid using around the eyes and sun exposure after applying, because it can cause sunspots on the skin.

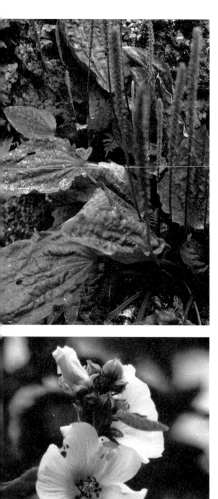

Plantain
(Plantago major)

- **Parts used.** The leaves and flower buds are cultivated at the end of spring.
- Plantain is grown in Europe and Asia. It blends well with chamomile, mint, thyme, sage and eucalyptus.
- Its soothing properties help to clear up respiratory ailments like cough, rough voice, snoring and pulmonary mucus. Gargle plantain to relieve an inflamed mouth or throat. This remedy is used as a syrup, tea or juice extracted from the fresh leaves and tincture.
- **Warning.** Use under strict medical supervision with children under 12 years of age and during pregnancy and breastfeeding.

A SOOTHING GARGLE

Boil previously ground plantain leaves, for 10 minutes.
Allow to steep, strain and cool.
You can use this mixture to gargle up to 3 times a day.

Marsh Mallow
(Althea officinalis)

- **Parts used.** Leaves, flowers and roots. The flowers are collected before they blossom and are used to make soothing syrups.
- This plant, native to the Mediterranean, grows wild in a wide area, stretching from Western

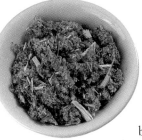

**SOOTHING
AN IRRITATED
THROAT**
Add a handful of
marsh mallow to
4 cups of water and
boil for 10 minutes.
Allow to steep and
strain. Drink 3
times a day,
sweetened to taste
with honey.

Europe to Siberia. Marsh mallow grows best in salty and cold areas.

• With its high content of mucilage, marsh mallow is used as a therapeutic remedy to relieve inflamed airways and for its soothing properties. It is also used externally to fight infected throats, pharyngitis and pulmonary ailments such as cough and bronchitis. It blends well with mullein and liquorice.

Horehound
(Marrubium vulgare)

• **Parts used.** The flowers are cultivated when they open and are dried placed on thin canopies.
• This plant, native to Central Asia, carries an aroma similar to apple. Its healing properties are good for fighting respiratory infections.
• Use as a remedy for excess phlegm and cough relief. Take 10 to 20 drops 3 times a day.
• **Warning.** Do not administer to children unless you consult your doctor. Not recommended during pregnancy or breastfeeding.

LIME
Relieves fevers and cold symptoms like irritated and watering eyes, sneezing, cough and sore throat. It has a fresh and slightly sweet citrus aroma.
Safety. It should be used in low concentration; and it's best to avoid direct sun after applying lime.

**MA HUANG
(EFEDRA)**
Anti-spasmodic. In China the branches are used –whole or crushed– to fight the common cold, especially symptoms of chills, headaches, achy body and a strong cough. This essential oil has antibacterial and antiviral properties. It blends well with primavera and thyme as a remedy against serious pulmonary ailments.
Safety. It shouldn't be used with other stimulants, if you are taking anti-depressive drugs or if you suffer from high blood pressure.

Yarrow
(Achillea millefolium)

<table>
<tr><td>

**TO FIGHT
A SLIGHT FEVER**

*Make an infusion
using 1 spoonful
of yarrow
and blue elderberry
in 1 cup of water,
allow to steep for
10 minutes and strain.
Drink up
to 4 cups daily.*

</td></tr>
</table>

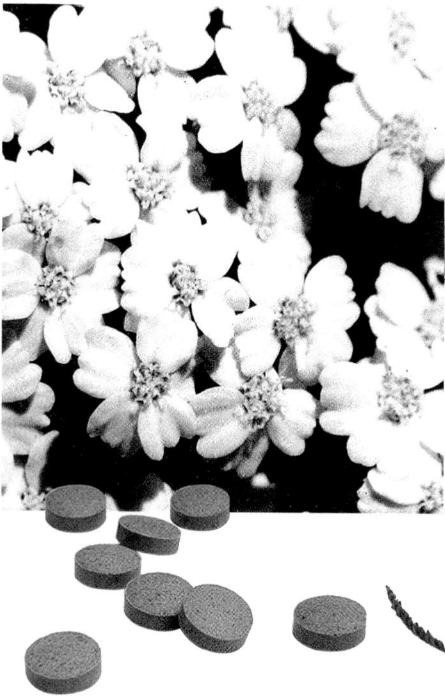

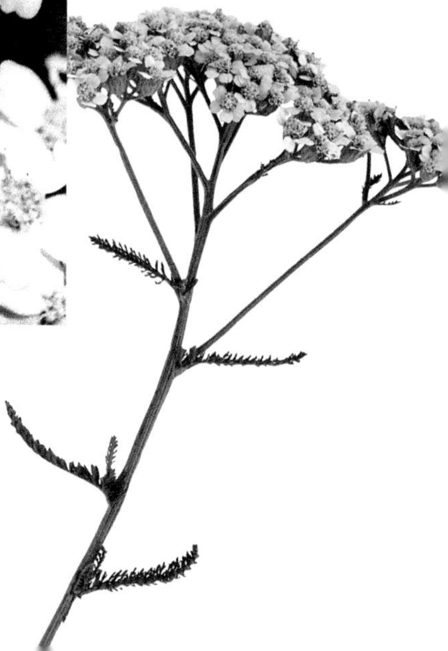

• **Parts used.** The flowers and leaves are harvested when blossoming and used to make infusions or teas. Yarrow has a slightly sweet and acidic taste that gives off a refreshing and toning sensation.

• This plant, native to the Mediterranean is today grown throughout Europe, North America and Asia. It has long been used for its anti-cold and anti-flu properties.

• Yarrow is good for its anti-inflammatory properties and for lowering fevers. Drink 3 cups a day.

• **Warning.** In high doses yarrow can cause dizziness and headaches. It increases the skin's sensitivity to the sun. It shouldn't be used in high doses during pregnancy because it stimulates the uterus.

Slippery elm
(Ulmus rubra)

• **Parts used.** The inner bark is used as a base for slippery elm tablets. It is also used in teas prepared from its powder.

• This tree native to North America has gained popularity in Europe, especially in Spain. Since the 70's the tree has been considered a plague because it has spread so widely that other tree species have not been able to grow in Europe and North America.

• Helps to fight colds and coughs. Native Americans have used the plant to sooth sore throats. It is used in capsules and infusions. It doesn't have any side effects.

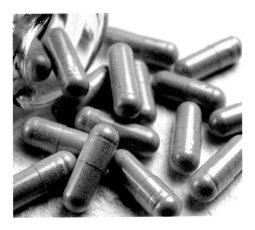

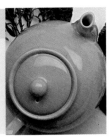

DRINK FOR A COMMON COLD

Mix a pinch of slippery elm bark powder in 1 cup of water and boil for 10 minutes. Allow to steep and strain. Drink cold.

ESSENTIAL OILS FROM A TO Z

MARJORAM
Relieves cold and flu symptoms. It has a pleasant aroma similar to almonds that calms headaches and a congested head caused by strong colds.
Safety. It is not recommended to use marjoram during pregnancy.

MINT
A nasal decongestant that improves breathing when the sinuses are stuffed up. Inhaling a few drops in a vapor solution can help to relieve and sooth discomfort caused by nasal congestion.
Safety. It is not recommended to use mint during pregnancy or breast-feeding, because it decreases the production of breast milk. It's recommended using mint in ointments or mixed with oils in low concentration to avoid skin irritation.

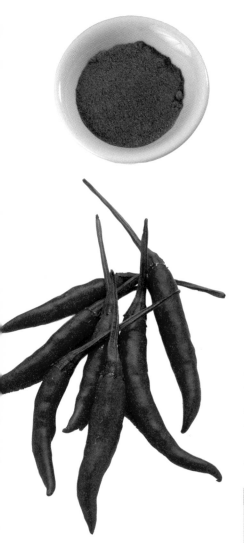

Cayenne
(Capsicum frutescens)

• **Parts used.** Fruit (fresh peppers) that are prepared in infusions, tinctures, salves and oils. The seeds should be removed because they can be toxic.

• Cayenne, which is native to India arrived to the West around 1,500 AD. Since then it has been cultivated throughout the world.

• The fruit causes sweating, which can be very good to fight fevers and chills. It is also a good remedy for throat problems like tonsillitis, laryngitis and strep throat.

• **Warning.** Do not use during pregnancy or breastfeeding. You should not touch your eyes, extremities or wounds with your hands after touching the fleshy inner part of fresh cayenne.

FOR A SORE THROAT

Add ¹/₂ spoonful of crushed cayenne to a small bowl of water. Place in a double boiler for 10 minutes. Next, strain and dilute 1 tablespoon in 1 cup of water. Take small sips to relieve a sore throat brought on by respiratory ailments and the common cold.

Liquorice
(Glycyrhiza glabra)

• **Parts used:** The roots are harvested in the fall and are rich in glycerol, which is 50 times sweeter than sucrose. Tinctures, syrups and candies are made with liquorice.
• Native to the Mediterranean and Central Asia, it has been cultivated in Europe since the 16th Century. In China it is known as "the great detoxifying root".
• It has strong soothing properties to alleviate pulmonary ailments and bronchitis. It is a great remedy for stomach ulcers.
• **Warning.** Should not be taken if you have high blood pressure, tumors, hormonal dependencies or diabetes. Do not take if you are taking any potassium depleting drugs.

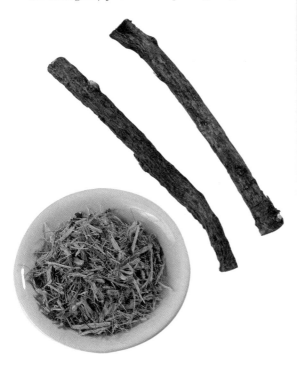

ESSENTIAL OILS FROM A TO Z

MYRRH
Pulmonary antiseptic and antitusive oil used to relieve symptoms related to bronchitis and a wet cough. This oil native to Ethiopia has a warm, sweet and resonating aroma. Myrrh is especially soothing for the lungs, chest pains and coughs. It doesn't have any side effects and can be used on children 2 years old and older.

PINE
Anti-cold and pulmonary anti-septic. Inhaled, it is a very good remedy for respiratory ailments especially if you are suffering from bronchitis, flu or sinus infection.
Safety. It is not recommended to use on children under 6 years old, pregnant women or during breastfeeding. It should not be used on patients with neurological diseases. In general, you should take care in using pine because excessive amounts can cause bronchial spasms.

Blue elderberry
(*Sambucus nigra*)

• **Parts used.** Fresh flowers, fruits, leaves and bark. The flowers are cultivated in the spring and fall, sun dried and stored in hermetic containers. The bark, cultivated in spring, is prepared as an infusion or used to make tinctures, syrups and creams. The ripe fruit, rich in vitamins A and C, is used to make beverages, served to prevent colds.

• Native to Europe and Asia, it is a shrub that grows in forests and along rivers and streams. In ancient times magic properties were attributed to the plant.

• It is an excellent antidote for respiratory illnesses. The flowers, when prepared in an infusion, induce sweating which helps get rid of the sickness. Blue elderberry relieves coughs that accompany the flu and soothes earaches.

• **Warning.** The fruit is toxic if not fully ripened.

CHILDREN WITH EAR INFECTIONS

Soak a handful of dried blue elderberry leaves in boiling water for 10 minutes. Wet a cotton ball from the steam released from the decoction and place in the ear. It can help to soothe pain caused by ear infections.

Thyme
(Thymus vulgaris)

• **Parts used.** The flowering tops and leaves are collected when the plant blossoms to make infusions, tinctures, syrups and oils.

• Thyme has antiseptic and soothing properties. It helps to ease bronchitis and throat and respiratory ailments. The flowers (rich in volatile oil) are a strong antiseptic and stimulate the body's defenses.

• **Warning.** You should avoid this remedy during pregnancy and if you have high blood pressure.

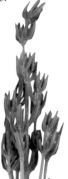

FOR NASAL CONGESTION
Prepare an infusion with a spoonful of dried thyme in 1 cup with boiling water. Allow to steep, strain and drink hot, up to 3 cups per day. This therapeutic infusion is good for getting rid of phlegm, mucus and nasal congestion.

ESSENTIAL OILS FROM A TO Z

RAVENSARA AROMATICA
Strong antibiotic. This essential oil with its refreshing aroma is especially recommended to treat the flu and common cold. The leaves are used to distill the essential oil (6 to 8 drops, applied on the body).

ROSEMARY
Stimulant, pain reliever, antispasmodic, anti-inflammatory and antiviral remedy. It's recommended mixing with mint and eucalyptus to treat respiratory problems and sinus infections. **Safety.** Rosemary shouldn't be used if you suffer from epilepsy, high blood pressure or are taking homeopathic treatments. Its use is not recommended if you are pregnant, because it stimulates the uterus.

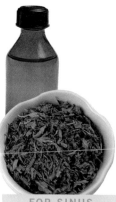

Golden root/rod
(*Solidago virga-aurea*)

• **Parts used.** Dried flowers are used to make beverages, syrups and tinctures.

• Native to Europe, Northern Asia, Africa and the Americas. It is also known as the "pagan herb"; it grows well in common gardens and as a wild plant.

• It helps to get rid of dead cells, detoxifying and purifying the body. It also helps to cure respiratory ailments.

• This herb works as an anti-inflammatory, antiseptic, sedative and sweat inducing remedy. It also helps to sooth inflamed mucous membranes.

• **Warning.** This remedy should not be used on children or during pregnancy and breastfeeding.

Wild Violet
(*Viola odorata*)

• **Parts used.** The flowers, leaves and roots are cultivated in the spring and used in syrups, tinctures and infusions. Wild violet

---

CHILDREN'S IMMUNE SYSTEM

To increase children's immune system use ravensara aromatica, an essential oil made with a special neutral vegetable oil that has similar effect but is better for children. Make this remedy by mixing 1 teaspoon of ravensara with 1 tablespoon of hazelnut oil. Use daily (once or twice per day) by massaging the oil on the chest, abdomen, arms and legs.

Use about 30 drops of oil for all the areas listed above.

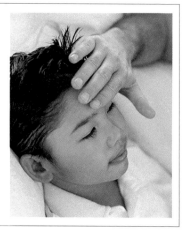

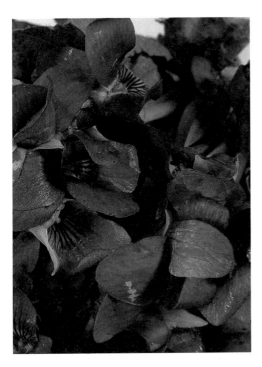

possesses a camphor-like and earthy aroma, similar to wood.

• An herb found in the Himalayas, it was used in Ancient Greece and Rome as a healing remedy.

• The remedy has expectorant properties, ideal to fight coughs, bronchitis and the common cold.

• **Warning.** In high doses this herb can be toxic and cause vomiting and nausea.

TO HELP GET RID OF PHLEGM

Wild violet roots possess healing properties that help to get rid of mucus. Place 1 spoonful of powder made from this plant's roots with 1 cup of water, let boil for 5 minutes and strain. Drink 2 or 3 cups per day.

ESSENTIAL OILS FROM A TO Z

SANDALWOOD

Pulmonary antiseptic that helps to soothe chest coughs. With its exotic, sweet and earthy aroma, it blends well with almond and lavender oil. You can mix sandalwood, almond oil, and lavender to make an ointment to treat children with colds and coughs by rubbing the salve on the chest and back.

TEA TREE

Tea tree is antiseptic and has an aroma of fresh wood. Not long ago it was discovered for its effects on respiratory ailments. Tea tree is ideal for fighting any type of infection due to the oil's double action property, which stimulates the immune system. It can be used on children under 2 years of age to help fight cold and flu symptoms. **Safety.** It should always be diluted because tea tree can irritate sensitive skin.

Fortyfying foods

Since ancient times food has been used as a natural remedy not only to prevent colds, flu and other common respiratory ailments but also to cure them. Over time, Western science has proven that a balanced and nutrient rich diet can help the body to fight against illnesses.

✚ The respiratory system is made up of a set of organs –the lungs, diaphragm and respiratory muscles– that transport oxygen to the body, which the cardiovascular system needs to function. The respiratory and cardiovascular systems, intrinsically related and delicate mechanisms, need essential nutrients to function properly. Many of these nutrients are antioxidants that help to protect the body against free radicals (unstable compounds that cause cellular and tissue damage) and help to strengthen your body's immune system.

WARNING
You should always consult your doctor before changing your diet.

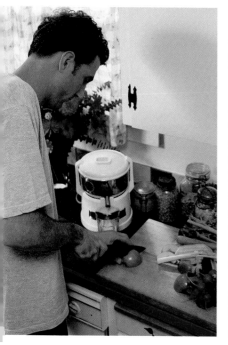

A diet that includes poli-unsaturated fats (unprocessed oils and seeds) stimulates our body's immune system, while a diet high in saturated fats (fats derived from red meats, butter, and dairy products) can increase your body's susceptibility to colds, flu, infections and other respiratory ailments.

It's proven that people who eat a high fiber and mono-unsaturated and poli-unsaturated fats rich diet based on vegetables and grains can fight bacteria and viruses better than those with a poor diet. Also, a balanced diet helps to improve your overall health.

Your body can not store vitamin C, therefore it must be consumed daily. It is a vitamin that helps to protect your body against illnesses. When our bodies lack vitamin C, our immune system weakens, opening the door to bacteria and viruses.

VITAMINS AND MINERALS

Our bodies need vitamins and minerals for specific uses in the body, especially for maintaining the body's immune system. Those of us eating a diet lacking vitamins and minerals tend to get colds and suffer from the flu (from slight to more serious symptoms).

Some of us with unhealthy daily habits need a higher intake of vitamins and minerals. Smokers, for example, need a higher amount of vitamin C than non-smokers. If you are managing a lot of stress, you need a higher daily intake of vitamins and minerals to stay healthy and to fight against respiratory infections.

In the following pages you will find a list of nutrients that are fundamental in fighting against colds and flu.

GARLIC

Garlic is a complete vegetable, providing proteins, sugars, calcium, phosphorus, iron and vitamins B, B_1 and C. Antibiotic properties found in garlic are a direct result of the allicin produced from raw, crushed garlic. Garlic helps to support the immune system, especially when eaten raw, but also cooked, it can help to fight against tonsillitis and sore throats.

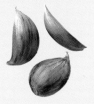

GARLIC BEVERAGE

Crush or finely chop 5 cloves of garlic. Mix with 5 spoonfuls of honey and add 1 cup of lukewarm water. Let sit 10 minutes and filter. This mixture can not be used the next day, so it's best to prepare the mixture fresh and have right away.

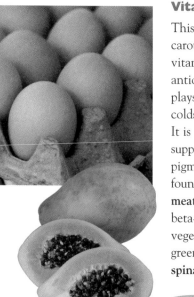

Vitamin A

This vitamin is converted from beta-carotene (which helps to support vitamin A). It is one of the principal antioxidants found in nature. Vitamin A plays an important role in preventing colds, flu and other respiratory illnesses. It is also known as retinol, which supports eye vision and generates pigments in the retina. Vitamin A is found in animal products such as **eggs**, **meat**, **milk**, **kidney** and **liver**; beta-carotene is found in fruits and vegetables that are orange, red and dark green like **sweet potatoes**, **yams**, **papaya**, **spinach**, **broccoli**, **carrots** and **squash**.

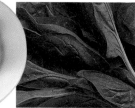

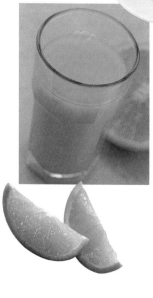

Vitamin C

Also known as ascorbic acid, it comprises, along with vitamins A and E, the three "antioxidants" found in nature. Vitamin C supports the production of white blood cells, the body's primary defender against infections. It also helps to protect your body against colds and other respiratory ailments. Your body does not store vitamin C, it is a water-soluble vitamin that your body excretes a short time after ingestion.

It's necessary to eat vitamin C rich foods or take the vitamin several times a day. Vitamin C works when accompanied by bioflavanoids (found in the citrus fruit rinds and white fleshy skin), calcium and magnesium. Fruits and vegetables rich in vitamin C include **brussels sprouts, cauliflower, strawberries, currants, kiwis, lemons, melons, oranges, green peppers, turnips** and **tomatoes.**

ONION

Onion is a wonderful source of minerals and micro-minerals –like sulfur– in addition to vitamins C and B and flavonoids, which are a strong antiviral remedy. This vegetable also has antibacterial properties and helps to relieve and treat ailments. You should eat at least 1/2 onion in your daily diet, alone or in salads, sauces or vegetable dishes.

ONION SYRUP

Dice 1 medium sized onion and mix with 3 spoonfuls of honey. Add water and cook in a double boiler. Let sit for 3 hours and then filter. You should drink between 5 to 10 spoonfuls throughout the day. This remedy can be given to children, but it's not recommended for children under 1 year of age.

ORANGES

Other than a high content of vitamin C, the oranges carry a number of fito-nutrients and antioxidants, including alpha-carotene and beta-carotene that protect the body. It helps the body to prevent and effectively fight against the common cold. Eating an abundant amount of oranges reduces cold symptoms and helps you get over illnesses quicker. Remember to eat the fleshy white skin below the rind that contains a high amount of bioflavanoids, which have a high concentrate of vitamin C.

ORANGE SALAD TO CURE A SORE THROAT

Peel 1 orange and cut it into slices. Add the orange slices to a leafy green salad, arugula for example, and if you like, add chopped sautéed onion. Add dressing to taste. Drinking orange juice is also a great way to increase your vitamin C intake (1 glass contains 90 mg of vitamin C).

ANTI-COLD BABY FOOD

Peel a large pumpkin; cut into pieces and steam. Next, blend in a blender so that the seeds are ground. Serve with a touch of olive oil. This is an excellent dish for children under the age of 5. Mashed pumpkin can be mixed with mashed summer squash (1 serving of 1/2 cup has approximately half the recommended daily intake of vitamin C for adults).

SQUASH/PUMPKIN

Helps to strengthen the immune system. Rich in beta-carotene and alpha-carotene (which gives its orange color) and antioxidants (vitamins C and E). Pumpkin seeds carry properties that help remove mucus from the lungs, bronchioles and throat. Because it is rich in antioxidants, it can help protect you against common colds and certain flu strains.

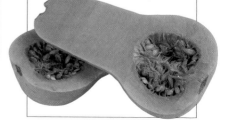

Vitamin E

It is also known as tocopherol and has four types: alfa, beta, gamma and delta.
A fat-soluble vitamin that acts as an antioxidant, it is important in the formation of red blood cells. Recent research has shown that vitamin E helps to strengthen the immune system and to prevent viral and bacterial attacks. Along with vitamin A, it helps to protect the lungs against pollution.

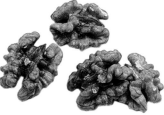

Warning. If you are taking an iron supplement, you should wait 8 hours before taking this vitamin. In high doses it can increase your blood pressure. Vitamin E is found in **wheat germ**, **broccoli**, **nuts** and other **seeds**, **olives**, **vegetable oils** (**corn**, **sunflower**, **soy**), **avocado**, **asparagus**, **spinach** and other **leafy green vegetables**.

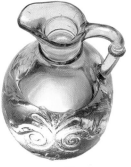

APPLE CIDER VINEGAR

Vinegar is produced when the acetic acid bacteria in alcohol change with the presence of oxygen. Over the centuries vinegar has not only been used as a condiment but also as a drink, preservative and natural remedy because it contains minerals and micro-elements like calcium, fluoride, magnesium, sodium, phosphorus, silica and potassium. Vinegar's curative properties are a result of the synergy between all of the ingredients, although the most important property is the antibacterial effect. For respiratory problems, apple cider vinegar can be used in vapor therapy to kill germs and to reduce bronchial mucus.

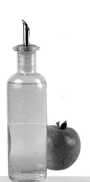

TO FIGHT AGAINST BRONCHITIS

Place 1 cup of cider vinegar in a bowl and add 2 cups of hot water. Inhale the steam between 5 to 10 minutes, taking in deep breaths with your head leaned over the bowl, a hand towel over your head to avoid losing steam. You can also use this mixture for compresses on the chest (tepid for chronic problems and cold for fevers).
To strengthen the respiratory system, you can prepare an infusion of apple cider vinegar and several spoonfuls of honey mixed together.

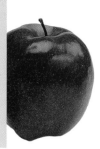

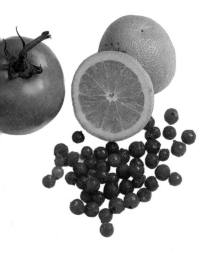

Vitamin P

Vitamin P's bioflavanoids enhance the action of vitamin C (so that the vitamin C is not destroyed by the air) and increase your resistance to infections. Vitamin P is not strictly speaking a vitamin. It is a classification of bioflavonoids, which refers to many different ingredients. It is also a powerful antioxidant that helps to neutralize damage caused by free radicals. Bioflavanoids are found in **citrus fruits**, **cherries**, **plums**, **berries**, **red grapes**, **green peppers**, **broccoli** and **tomatoes**.

Vitamin B$_2$

B$_2$ is a water-soluble vitamin that supports the energy metabolism and the immune system, keeping the mucous membranes that coat the respiratory and digestive systems healthy. It's a vital vitamin for our bodies' growth and cell reproduction, in particular to produce red blood cells. It helps the body to absorb iron and in the assimilation of vitamins A and B$_1$. Natural sources are **meats, dairy products, wholewheat flour, wheat germ, green veggies, dried fruits** and **yeast**.

HONEY

This sweet substance may act as a general antibiotic and carries inhibitors that may fight bacteria and avoid infections. It helps to relieve cold symptoms and soothe irritations. It can be used as a daily supplement. Because of its sweet and delicious taste, it is good for children. Due to honey's high sugar content, be sure to brush your teeth after eating it.

Safety. Children under 1 year of age should not consume honey, because the intestine is not fully developed to digest this food.

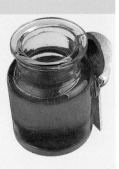

Vitamin B_6

Of all of the B complex vitamins, B_6 is crucial for the immune system's health, because it plays an important role in boosting the production of antibodies that our bodies use to fight diseases. It helps to prevent infections (among those, respiratory illnesses) and is a vital part of the immune system's functioning. It is also necessary in the absorption of B_{12} (in general all B complex vitamins work together and are found in the same types of foods). It is also fundamental in increasing the levels of serotonin (a natural brain chemical), that reduces the risk of aches and pains in the body. This is why B_6 is an effective vitamin for pains and symptoms related to premenstrual syndrome. It is water-soluble, and cooking can destroy up to 90 percent of this vitamin found in foods.

It's suggested that you eat fresh or undercooked foods for B_6 intake. **Seeds**, **whole grains**, **beans**, **bananas**, **nuts** and **potatoes** are all rich in B_6.

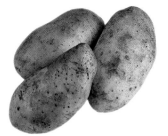
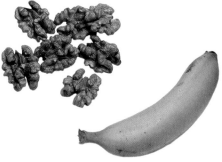

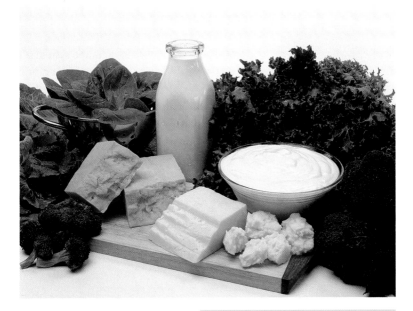

LENTILS

Other than being a folic acid rich food, lentils are also high in B_1, B_2, B_3 and B_6 vitamins. They are also a great source of protein, especially if prepared with rice. They are rich in iron, calcium, zinc and potassium. A dish prepared with lentils is a very complete and beneficial food, because it helps to fortify the immune system.

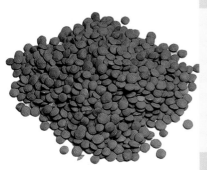

HEALTHY SALAD
**For a delicious
and health supporting fresh salad**
Slice 2 carrots and 1 onion.
Add 2 diced garlic cloves, lentils,
bay leaf and 1 teaspoon of thyme. Cover
and cook for 15 minutes on a low heat.
Drain and remove the bay leaf. Put the
lentils in the refrigerator to cool. Dress
with olive oil, salt and pepper. It can be
served at room temperature.

Folic acid

Folic acid is a B complex vitamin that boosts the immune system and helps to prevent respiratory illnesses, especially colds and flu. A folic acid rich diet should include plenty of **whole grains**, **beans**, **fruits** and **green leafy vegetables**.

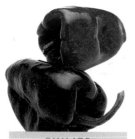

CHILIES AND PEPPERS

Strengthen the immune system and act as a natural pain reliever. The plant's active substance, capsicum (which gives peppers their hot, spicy flavor) also stimulates the immune system. They are also rich in vitamin C and carotene. Eating peppers as part of your daily diet can aid in reducing and shortening your illness. A medium pepper contains three times more than the daily-recommended intake of vitamin C for adults.

Safety. It's important to avoid cayenne pepper in infusions and gargling during pregnancy and breastfeeding.

Zinc

Is an essential mineral needed to support your metabolism and it has antiviral properties that help to relieve colds. It supports the immune system, because it stimulates the division and development of the cells that defend the body. It helps the body's natural ability to shield against bacterial infections. Some studies have shown that diets which include a zinc supplement reduce the incidence of respiratory infections. Zinc is found in: **red meat (veal, pork** and **lamb), peanuts, beans, seafood, whole cereals, egg yolks, brewers yeast, liver, sunflower seeds** and **pumpkin**.

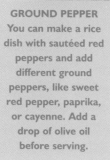

GROUND PEPPER
You can make a rice dish with sautéed red peppers and add different ground peppers, like sweet red pepper, paprika, or cayenne. Add a drop of olive oil before serving.

Iron

Essential for the support of the protein hemoglobin and red blood cells. An iron deficiency can cause a drop in your immune system. Children who have a diet lacking iron tend to get sick more often. They tend to be weak, get exhausted and frequently catch the flu and colds. Children and teenagers who have a poor diet often suffer from anemia caused by low hemoglobin in the blood brought on by an iron deficiency. The best sources for iron are **liver, lean red meat, tuna** and **salmon, fortified cereals, whole grains, eggs** (the **yolks** are rich in iron), **dried fruits, nuts, seeds** and **leafy green vegetables**.

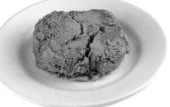

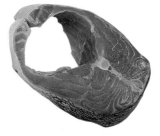

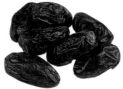

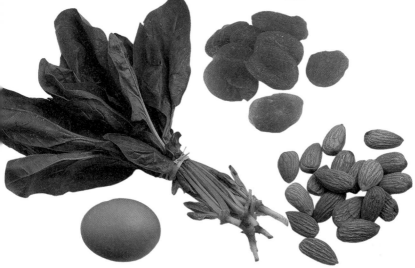

index

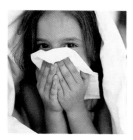